COOK BOOK

FOR

CANCER PATIENTS

Sustaining strength with cancer-friendly dishes: Healing recipes, Nourishing meals, Post-treatment recipe guide, Meal plans and Nutrient-rich dishes for survivors

Brandon Oliver

TABLE OF CONTENTS

Brandon Oliver

INTRODUCTION

In the world of heartwarming cookbooks for cancer patients, we're not just mixing pots and pans in this kitchen companion. We create a symphony of flavors tailored to the unique needs of people bravely facing cancer. Think of this cookbook as your ally in the kitchen, a friend that provides comfort and flavor during your arduous journey. This is correct! Cancer poses its own challenges, especially in the food sector. That's why we've prepared a variety of recipes that go beyond flavor. These recipes are created with love, care and an understanding of the culinary transformation that accompanies healing. From easy-to-swallow snacks to creative twists that keep sugar and fat in check, our recipes are culinary hugs designed to bring joy and nutrition to your meal. This cookbook isn't just about food. It's a celebration of resilience and a reminder that even in difficult times, a well-prepared meal can be a source of strength and comfort. So grab your oars, put on your favorite apron and join us on this delicious journey where each recipe tells a story of care, hope and the amazing power of delicious food. Welcome to the kitchen. Let's cook positive dishes!

CHAPTER 1

UNDERSTANDING NUTRITION IN CANCER PATIENTS

Understanding nutrition is an important consideration for people navigating the complex cancer journey. For cancer patients, the connection between nutrition and well-being is even deeper. It goes beyond simple nutrition and plays an important role in maintaining overall health, managing the side effects of treatments and potentially influencing the course of the disease. Recognizing the complex interplay between diet and cancer requires recognizing the unique challenges patients face. The effects of cancer and cancer treatment on the body's metabolic processes can lead to changes such as changes in appetite, weight loss, or nutritional deficiencies. Therefore, it is important to understand the nutritional requirements to effectively address these issues.

In this context, the role of a balanced individual diet cannot be overemphasized. This is intended not only to meet calorie requirements but also to provide a variety of nutrients that contribute to the body's resistance. Adequate intake of protein, vitamins, minerals and other essential elements is essential to support the body's ability to cope with disease and treatment needs. Additionally, nutritional issues go beyond macro and micronutrient levels. For example, hydration is important for managing dehydration, which is common during cancer treatment. Hydration plays an important role in supporting various body functions and reducing potential side effects.

Understanding nutrition in cancer patients also includes addressing specific nutritional issues related to treatment. For example, specific nutritional strategies may be needed to manage nausea, taste changes, or difficulty swallowing. Adopting a flexible and adaptive approach to diet can significantly improve patients' quality of life and maintain nutritional status. It is equally important to recognize that nutritional needs may evolve along the cancer trajectory. Regular assessments, in collaboration with your doctor, will allow you to adjust your meal plan as your needs and response to treatment change. This dynamic approach reflects the ongoing dialogue between nutrition and the complexity of disease.

In fact, understanding nutrition for cancer patients goes beyond traditional nutritional advice. This includes a holistic understanding of the patient's unique situation while recognizing the symbiotic relationship between nutrition and overall well-being. With this understanding, healthcare providers can optimize the nutritional status of cancer patients, increase recovery, and support a holistic approach to treatment.

The role of nutrition in cancer treatment

The role of nutrition in cancer treatment is a multifaceted and essential part of comprehensive care. This goes beyond simple supportive measures and becomes a key aspect of addressing disease challenges and therapeutic interventions. Nutrition plays an important role in maintaining the overall health of people receiving cancer treatment. The impact of the disease and its treatment on the body's physiological processes requires a strategic and individualized approach to nutritional support. Adequate nutrition is the basis for addressing issues such as weight loss, maintaining energy levels and reducing the risk of malnutrition.

Nutrition is also closely related to the body's ability to tolerate and respond to cancer treatment. Chemotherapy, radiation and other treatments can cause significant stress on the body, affecting the immune system, metabolism and gastrointestinal function. A well-designed and coordinated nutritional plan can increase the body's tolerance, reduce treatment-related side effects, and optimize the effectiveness of therapeutic interventions. In addition to its physiological effects, nutrition also plays an important role in improving the quality of life of people receiving cancer treatment. Addressing issues such as loss of appetite, changes in taste and diet is important to improve psychological well-being and reduce the emotional toll that comes with the cancer journey. The dynamic nature of cancer treatment requires continuous evaluation and adjustment of nutritional strategies. Healthcare professionals work with patients to monitor nutritional status and ensure meal plans evolve based on treatment response and changing needs. This personalized approach recognizes the uniqueness of each person's cancer experience and tailors nutritional intervention accordingly.

Nutrition is a very important factor in the fight against cancer. A healthy diet can help cancer patients get all the nutrients their bodies need to stay healthy during the necessary treatment period. It also boosts immunity and reduces inflammation. In addition, a healthy diet helps maintain energy levels so you can better cope with physical activity and other treatments.

Brandon Oliver

Brandon Oliver

CHAPTER 2

NUTRITIOUS FOOD FOR CANCER PATIENTS

There are several types of nutrients that are particularly beneficial for cancer patients. For example, protein helps repair cells damaged by radiation or chemotherapy, while omega-3 fatty acids fight inflammation caused by tumors. Vitamins A and C strengthen immunity, and zinc helps protect against infection. Magnesium helps you relax and reduce stress levels. Iron helps prevent anemia. Antioxidants like beta-carotene fight free radicals that damage cells.

1. Proteins

Protein is essential for cell renewal and growth, making it a very important part of a cancer patient's diet. Protein can be found in foods such as lean meat, eggs, dairy products and legumes. Protein shakes and other supplements can be good options for people who have difficulty chewing or swallowing.

2. Fat

Fat is an important source of energy for cancer patients receiving chemotherapy. Fats also provide essential fatty acids that help maintain cell integrity and immunity and reduce inflammation in the body. Healthy sources of fat include avocados, nuts, seeds and fatty fish such as salmon and mackerel.

3. Carbohydrates

Carbohydrates provide energy to every cell in the body and provide important vitamins and minerals for health. Whole grains such as oats and quinoa are excellent sources of carbohydrates, along with fruits, vegetables and legumes such as beans and lentils. All of these foods should be included in the diet of cancer patients during chemotherapy or other treatment courses. Foods that cancer patients should avoid

It is also important to note that people undergoing cancer treatment should avoid certain foods completely. This includes meats that have been processed, examples are sausages and bacon. High-fat dairy products such as butter and cheese; Fried foods such as French fries and doughnuts; refined carbohydrates such as white bread or pasta; Sweets, such as candies or cookies; Foods with artificial colors or preservatives; alcohol; cigarette; And excessive amounts of caffeine. All of these substances should be excluded from the patient's diet, as they can interfere with recovery time and cause additional health complications.

Expert nutritional advice for cancer patients

Healthy eating is important to fight cancer. The best way to approach this is to consult with your doctor or a registered dietitian who specializes in cancer nutrition. They can make recommendations about foods to eat and avoid based on your specific needs to ensure your body has all the nutrients it needs to recover. Also note that the role of nutrition in cancer treatment goes beyond basic diet. It is an essential part of a holistic treatment approach and contributes to the overall well-being, resilience and treatment outcomes of those being treated. Nutrition, as a supportive and dynamic part of cancer treatment, emphasizes the importance of a comprehensive and individualized approach to meet the diverse needs of patients throughout their cancer treatment journey.

Nutritional information for cancer patients

Dietary considerations for cancer patients include a nuanced approach that goes beyond conventional nutritional advice. Recognizing the unique challenges associated with cancer and its treatment, personalized nutritional strategies play an important role in supporting overall well-being and managing treatment-related side effects.

Balanced diet: Ensuring a balanced and varied diet is important for cancer patients. Adequate intake of protein, carbohydrates, healthy fats, vitamins and minerals supports the body's nutritional needs and contributes to overall health and resilience.

Caloric and protein intake: Maintaining adequate caloric intake is especially important for patients who have lost weight or need increased energy. Adequate protein intake is important for maintaining muscle mass and promoting recovery.

Hydration: Good hydration is important for managing treatment-related side effects and supporting various body functions. Cancer treatments, such as chemotherapy, can sometimes lead to dehydration, making fluid intake an important issue.

High-fiber foods: Including high-fiber foods in your diet can help manage constipation, a common side effect of certain cancer treatments. Fruits and vegetables also whole grains are good sources of dietary fiber.

Adapt to changes in taste: Cancer treatment can change your taste and make certain foods more appealing. Experimenting with different flavors and textures, using herbs and spices, and trying new recipes make your food delicious.

Treatment for nausea: Nausea is a common side effect of cancer treatment. Choosing soft, easily digestible foods, eating smaller and more frequent meals, and avoiding strong smells can help control nausea.

Individualized planning: Nutrition plans should be individualized, recognizing that each patient's cancer experience is unique. Factors such as the type of cancer, treatment options, and personal preferences affect nutritional needs.

Supplements: In some cases, supplements may be recommended to address specific nutritional deficiencies or to support overall nutritional status. However, all supplements should be discussed with your healthcare provider to ensure compatibility with your ongoing treatment.

Collaboration with healthcare professionals: Effective communication and collaboration with oncologists, nutritionists and other healthcare professionals is essential. Regular assessment of nutritional status and adjustment of meal plans based on treatment response contribute to a comprehensive treatment approach.

CHAPTER 3

MANAGING SIDE EFFECTS OF CANCER TREATMENT

Cancer treatments, such as radiotherapy or chemotherapy, can cause side effects such as:

• Disease

• Vomiting

• Constipation

• Diarrhea

• Fatigue

• Loss of appetite

• Taste changes

• Difficulty swallowing

• Mouth inflammation and pain

• Metallic or bitter taste

Dietary guidelines for cancer patients
Healthy eating habits are very important for cancer patients during and after cancer treatment. Adequate nutrition provides the following benefits:

• You feel better

• Maintain a healthy weight

• Better recovery

• Strengthen your immune system

You may be able to tolerate the side effects of treatment better.

Here are some recommendations for what to eat to manage the side effects of cancer treatment:

Nausea and vomiting

• Eat soft, easily digestible food.

• Eat small meals instead of large meals throughout the day.

• Eat citrus fruits like oranges, grapefruit and limes.

• Ginger contains bioactive compounds such as paradol, shogaol and gingerol that help with nausea.

• Eat food that have been dry examples of such food are dry crackers and toast.

Constipation

• Increase your dietary fiber intake. Good sources include fruits, vegetables and oats.

• Drink a lot of water.

Diarrhea

• BRAT diet - bananas, rice, apples, toast. These soft foods are better for your digestive system.

• If you are dehydrated, drink clear broth or water containing electrolytes to stay hydrated.

Loss of appetite

After cancer treatment, you may feel tired all the time and lose your appetite. However, nutrient intake is essential for optimal recovery. Instead of eating large meals, eat small meals 4-5 times a day and choose nutritious foods.

Change of taste

• If you can't really taste the food, it can be difficult to eat it.

• Try adding considerable amount of spices to your meals.

• Eat your favorite foods when you don't feel nauseous.

• If your tongue tastes metallic or bitter, try sugar-free lemon, gum or peppermint drops.

Problems swallowing or chewing

• Choose soft foods such as porridge, porridge, soft-boiled eggs and boiled cereals. You can also add high-calorie drinks like smoothies or milkshakes.

• Avoid spicy, hard, tough and acidic foods.

• Consider using a straw when drinking soups and drinks.

Mouth inflammation and pain

• Choose foods that are comforting to the palate, such as well-prepared foods such as ice cream, frozen fruit, yogurt, smoothies, and casseroles.

• Avoid acidic or spicy foods such as tomatoes and oranges.

• Eat room temperature or cold foods rather than hot foods.

What should cancer patients eat?
A balanced diet with the right nutrition is always important.

• Eat lots of fiber and protein.

• By adding the right fats rich in omega-3 fatty acids in the meal.

• Remember, Drink plenty of water.

Avoid the following foods:

• Alcohol

• Fried or fried foods

• Ultra-processed foods like chips and junk food

• Refined carbohydrates such as white pasta, bread, rice, etc.

• Raw eggs, fish, shellfish, meat and poultry

• Unpasteurized milk or cheese

• Raw foods like sushi and raw beans

CHAPTER 4

STOCKING A CANCER-FRIENDLY KITCHEN FOR CANCER PATIENTS

Providing food to cancer patients requires careful selection of foods that support their nutritional needs, mitigate side effects of treatment, and promote overall well-being. Creating a nutrient-rich environment in the kitchen can improve a patient's ability to maintain a healthy diet during and after cancer treatment.

When stocking a cancer patents kitchen, consider the following components:

Fresh fruits and vegetables: Provide colorful fruits and vegetables rich in vitamins, minerals and antioxidants. People with digestive problems should choose foods that are easy to digest, such as bananas, melons and cooked vegetables.

Lean protein: Lean protein sources include poultry, fish, tofu and legumes. Protein is essential for maintaining muscle mass and supporting the body during healing.

Whole grains: Choosing whole grains such as brown rice, quinoa, oats, and whole grain bread can provide long-lasting energy and dietary fiber that aids digestion.

Healthy fats fruits: By eating healthy fats like olive oil, nuts, seeds and avocados. These fats are essential for overall health and can help increase calorie intake in people concerned about weight loss.

Low-fat milk or dairy alternatives: For those who can tolerate dairy, include low-fat options or consider dairy alternatives such as almond milk or soy milk.

Hydration options: Offer fluids such as water, herbal teas, and clear broth to keep your child hydrated, especially during treatments that can cause dehydration.

Easy-to-eat foods: Keep easy-to-digest foods on hand in case you lose your appetite or have indigestion. This can be crackers, plain rice or plain soup.

Ginger and Anger: This can help control nausea, a common side effect of cancer treatment. Ginger tea or peppermint candies can have a calming effect.

Comfort foods: Include comfort foods that are easy to prepare, enjoyable and provide psychological support during difficult times.

Meal Replacement Surgery: When eating solid foods is difficult, eating meal replacement shakes or smoothies can provide adequate nutrition.

Flexible Freezing Options: Keep a variety of frozen fruits, vegetables and pre-cooked proteins in the freezer for convenience and to reduce food waste.

Food Storage Containers: Invest in storage containers to distribute and store food for easy access and organization, especially during low energy times.

Collaboration with healthcare providers: We work closely with healthcare providers and nutritionists to tailor the cuisine to the individual patient's needs, taking into account dietary restrictions and preferences.

By carefully stocking the kitchen with nutritious, easily digestible, and convenient options, caregivers and patients can create an environment that promotes healthy eating during cancer treatment. Regular communication with healthcare providers ensures that nutritional choices are aligned with the patient's specific health goals and treatment plan.

Eat well during cancer treatment

During treatment, the clinical nutritionist may recommend certain foods to help you eat more calories, eat more protein, or eat more comfortably. Some of these foods may seem like unhealthy choices. It is important to remember that the time period for eating this way is very short. Once the side effects disappear and your appetite returns to normal, you can stop eating foods that you consider unhealthy. A clinical nutritionist can help you find the meal plan that's best for you.

Tips for eating and drinking

In the cause of treatment, you might have good days and bad days when it comes to eating. Large meals can seem heavy or unappealing. This can be caused by loss of appetite (wanting to eat less than usual) or early satiety (feeling full soon after you start eating). The following suggestions will help you get the most out of your meals.

• Eat small, frequent meals. For example, instead of three main meals, eat six to eight times a day.

• Eat every few hours. Don't wait until you're hungry.

• Place smaller portions on a salad plate instead of a plate.

• Drink high-calorie hot chocolate, fruit juice and honey.

• Avoid low-calorie beverages such as water, coffee, tea, and diet drinks. Make double milks and milkshakes using the recipes in the recipe section.

• Make sure you can eat the foods you like at home, on the go and at work.

• Eat your best foods at any time. For example, eat breakfast (such as pancakes or an omelet) for lunch or dinner.

• Add different colors and textures to food to make it more appealing.

• Create a better dining experience by dining with family or friends in a pleasant and comfortable environment.

• Prepare food that smells good, such as baking bread or frying bacon.

Ways to add good amount of protein to your diet

Your body needs the right of calories and protein to function properly. Your doctor even your nutritionist may tell you to for the main time increase the amount of protein in your diet. Maybe you have recently had surgery perhaps an injury, eating good amount of protein can help with healing. Some of the ways that will help you increase right amount of protein in your diet are:

•   Eat protein-rich foods such as chicken, fish, pork, beef, lamb, eggs, milk, cheese, beans, nuts or nut butters, and soy products.

• Drink skim milk and use it in recipes that call for milk or water, such as quick puddings, cocoa, omelets, and pancake mix. To make double milk, combine 1 bag (about 1 cup) of skimmed milk powder and 1 quart of whole milk in a blender, store in the refrigerator.

• Use double milk or a ready-to-eat topping (such as Verzecker on hot or cold breakfast cereal).

• Add cheese and ground cooked meat to an omelet or quiche.

• Add unflavored protein powder to creamy soups, mashed potatoes, smoothies and casseroles.

• Snack crackers with cheese or nut butter (peanut butter, cashew butter, almond butter, etc.).

• Spread nut butter on apples, bananas and celery.

• Try the cheese curds and apple slices drizzled with honey.

• Blend nut butter into shakes or smoothies.

• Snack on nuts, sunflower or pumpkin seeds.

• Add nuts and seeds to breads, muffins, pancakes, cookies and waffles.

• Try hummus with pita bread. Use hummus as a spread on sandwiches or add a spoonful to a salad.

• Add cooked meat to soups, stews and salads.

• Add wheat germ, hazelnuts, chia seeds, or flaxseed flour to breakfast cereals, casseroles, and yogurt.

• Choose Greek yogurt over plain yogurt.

• Try egg desserts like cake, pudding, custard and cheesecake.

• Add eggs or protein to custard, pudding, quiche, pancake batter, toast, scrambled eggs or scrambled eggs.

• Melt the cheese over the burgers and breaded patties.

• Add beans, peas, tofu, boiled eggs, nuts, seeds and cooked meat or fish to the salad.

• You can use pasteurized bone broth in making your soups and stews.

Ways to add good amount of protein to your diet

The following suggestions will help you eat more calories. This may seem contrary to what you already know about healthy eating. However, the most important thing during treatment and while you are healing is to eat enough calories and protein.

• Avoid labeling foods and beverages as low-fat, fat-free, or diet. Snack on dried fruit, nuts or dried seeds. Add to hot cereal, ice cream and salads.

• Drink fruit juice in a fruit cocktail.

• Add butter, oil or oil to potatoes, rice and pasta. Also add it to cooked vegetables, sandwiches, toast and hot cereal.

• Add cream cheese or nut butter to toast or bagels or spread over vegetables.

• Spread cream cheese, jam and peanut butter on crackers.

• Try adding jelly or honey to bread or crackers.

• Mix the finely chopped fruits with the jam and put them on top of the ice cream or cake.

• Snack on tortilla chips with guacamole or sour cream.

• Add sour cream, coconut milk, half and half or heavy cream to mashed potatoes, cookies and brownies recipes. It can also be added to pancake batter, gravies, sauces, soups and casseroles.

• Sprinkle cheese or cream on the baked potatoes.

• Top cake, waffles, French toast, fruit, pudding and hot chocolate with whipped cream.

• Drizzle cream sauce or drizzle olive oil on vegetables or pasta before eating.

• Use mayonnaise, creamy salad dressing or aioli on salads, sandwiches and vegetable dips.

• Mix yogurt with granola or top it with ice cream or fruit. Use granola in cookies, muffins, and bread dough.

• Glazed or unglazed cake with sweet condensed milk. Combining condensed milk and peanut butter adds more calories and flavor.

• Add croutons to the salad.

• Add the filling to the plate as a garnish.

• Try a homemade cocktail. Try our shake recipes in our recipe section. You can also drink high-calorie, high-protein drinks like Carnation Breakfast Essentials or Zorgen.

• Add avocado as a spread to smoothies, soups, salads, omelets and toast.

• Add good amount of mayonnaise also sour cream to salads, you can use it as a spread on sandwiches any time.

In general, nutritional issues in cancer patients require a holistic and individualized approach that takes into account the dynamic nature of the disease and treatment. By meeting nutritional needs and addressing treatment concerns, a well-designed meal plan can make a significant contribution to the overall quality of life and well-being of people battling cancer.

Brandon Oliver

CHAPTER 5

MANAGEMENT OF SYMPTOMS AND SIDE EFFECTS THROUGH DIET

This section provides some tips that may help you.

• Loss of appetite

• Constipation

• Diarrhea (soft or liquid stools)

• Dry mouth

• Mouth or throat pain

• Taste changes

• Early satiety

• Disease

• Fatigue

Tell your doctor or nurse if you have any of the above problems before following these tips. Dietary changes can help, but medication may be needed to better control side effects. If you have been given drugs prescriptions, take it as been directed by your healthcare provider.

Appetite loss

Anorexia refers to a decreased appetite or desire to eat. This is a common side effect of cancer treatment. There may be certain times of the day when your appetite improves so you can eat more. If so, try to use this time to eat as much as possible. For ideas on how to get the most out of meals and snacks, see the Calorie and Protein Intake section of this resource.

Sometimes you're not hungry at all. If so, make a meal plan. For example, instead of waiting until you're hungry eat every two hours. Setting an alarm for yourself can help.

Constipation

Constipation is one of the major problems that make bowel movements difficult. If you are constipated, have a bowel movement:

• It's too difficult

• Too small

• It's hard to go out

• Less than usual

Constipation can be caused by a variety of factors, including diet, activity and lifestyle. Some chemotherapy and pain relievers can cause constipation. Here are some ways to manage constipation through diet:

Eat more fiber-rich foods

Fiber is important because it increases the volume of the stool in the stool. It increases the elimination of waste from the body system. Add fiber to your diet with one meal. Drink plenty of fluids to avoid gas and bloating. Examples of high-fiber foods include:

• Fruits

• Vegetables

• Bran cake

• Whole grains such as pasta, bread and brown rice

• Nuts and seeds

Drink a lot of water

Try to drink at least 8-10 glasses of fluids a day, this helps keep your stool soft.

Motion Exercise also helps with constipation. Do light physical activity (walking, climbing stairs slowly, etc.) to keep food moving through the digestive system. Before you engage on physical activities seek the counsel of your doctor.

Diarrhea

Diarrhea – frequent passage of soft, watery stools. This helps food pass through the intestines quickly. In this case, water and nutrients are not properly absorbed by the body. Diarrhea can be caused by:

• Chemotherapy

• Radiotherapy

• Stomach or intestinal surgery

• Approximate

• Difficulty digesting milk and milk products

• There are too many sugar alcohols, such as sorbitol or mannitol, found in sugar-free snacks.

• Other food sensitivities

Consult your doctor before using any of the suggestions below to control diarrhea. Drink a lot of water

Drink at least 8 to 10 glasses (8-ounce glasses) of fluid a day. It helps replace water and nutrients lost due to diarrhea. Try it:

• Fruit juice, juice mixed with water

• Fragrance-free pediatric medication

• Coconut water

• Electrolyte tablets that can be added to water, such as Nuun

• Electrolyte powder mixed with water as a drop

• Water containing electrolytes such as helices

• Decaffeinated soda. Leave it open for a few minutes before drinking to reduce gas.

Dry mouth

Dry mouth can occur due to:

• Chemotherapy

• Radiotherapy

• Approximate

• Head and neck surgery

• Infection

• Other health problems

Dry mouth can also cause cavities. This helps protect your teeth from decay by producing less saliva. Dental hygiene (taking care of your mouth) is very important when you have dry mouth. Avoid alcohol-based mouthwash. Instead, rinse your mouth with a mixture of 1 teaspoon of baking soda and 1 teaspoon of salt in 1 liter (4 cups) of warm water. Rinse your mouth with this mouthwash every two hours.

A dry mouth can make eating difficult. Some foods may be difficult to chew or swallow. The type of food you eat changes. Choose foods that are moist, soft in texture and easy to swallow. Avoid dry or rough foods. Drink plenty of fluids throughout the day. Sipping liquid between bites while eating makes it easier to chew and swallow food.

Sore mouth or throat

Mouth and throat ulcers can result from certain chemotherapy treatments and radiation treatment to the head or neck.

Mouth or throat pain makes eating difficult. The way you eat is changing. Here are some tips to prevent oral irritation:

• Cook food until soft and tender.

• Cut food into small, easy-to-chew pieces.

• Rinse your mouth often. Try making a mouthwash with 1 teaspoon of salt, 1 teaspoon of baking soda, and 1 liter (4 cups) of warm water. If this does not help, ask your doctor for recommendations on other mouthwashes.

• Use a straw when drinking. This will prevent the liquid from reaching the sore mouth.

• Brush your teeth and tongue if your doctor or dentist says it's okay.

• Drink more fluids to keep your mouth clean. If you have a sore mouth or throat, it may help to eat soft, bland, warm or cold foods. Avoid foods that aggravate the pain, such as dry foods, spicy, salty, sour and acidic foods.

Change of taste

The sense of taste can be affected by chemotherapy, radiotherapy and certain medicines.

Taste is composed of five basic senses: salty, sweet, umami, bitter and sour. Taste changes vary from person to person. The most common change is a bitter, metallic taste in the mouth. Sometimes you don't even taste the food at all. These changes usually disappear after treatment. Proper oral care is essential to prevent taste changes. This can be done by brushing your teeth and tongue (if your doctor or dentist says it's okay) and drinking more fluids. You can also make your own mouthwash by mixing 1 teaspoon of baking soda and 1 teaspoon of salt in 1 liter (4 cups) of warm water. Use mouthwash regularly throughout the day (before and after meals). If the food seems tasteless

• Change the texture of the food. For example, you might prefer baked mashed potatoes.

• Try changing the temperature of the food. Some foods are better cold or at room temperature.

• Select and make a preparation of foods that look and also smell good.

Use more spices and flavors if they do not cause discomfort. e.g:

• Add sauces and condiments (such as soy sauce or ketchup) to food.

• Marinate meat or meat substitutes in salad dressing, fruit juice or other dressings.

• Use onions or garlic to season vegetables or meat.

• Add herbs (rosemary, basil, oregano, mint, etc.) to food.

• Try mixing fruit into a milkshake or yogurt.

• Try to eat sour and spicy foods. This will help improve your taste buds.

 Enjoy a variety of delicious snacks as you eat. For example, try this:

• Cottage cheese and pineapple.

• Canned fruit and yogurt.

• Grilled cheese and tomato juice.

When you have that bitter even metallic taste in your mouth

• Rinse your mouth with water before eating.

• If the meat tastes spicy, marinate it in sauce or fruit juice or squeeze a little lemon juice before eating. Do this only if your mouth does not hurt.

• Add meat alternatives (dairy, soy, etc.) to protein.

• Use plastic containers.

• Try mints or sugar-free gum.

• Avoid canned foods (sauce, soups, etc.). Instead, choose items that come in glass or plastic bottles or boxes.

When food tastes too sweet

•Add some salt to your food.

• Dilute sugary drinks with water.

• If everything is sweet, try eating more acidic foods, such as foods with lemon.

If the taste or smell of food is different from usual

• Avoid strong smelling foods. Beef and fish have the strongest odors, so it is recommended to eat poultry, eggs and dairy products.

• When cooking, open the lids of pots and pans away from your body to eliminate odors.

• If the smell of cooking bothers you, open the window while cooking.

• Let the food cool before eating, room temperature or cold foods have less odor than warm foods.

• Experiment with different combinations of spices and foods, including adding sauces to food and changing the temperature and texture of foods.

• If your mouth doesn't hurt, try eating grated foods (like lemon or citrus slices) to stimulate your taste buds.

• Rinse your mouth before and after meals.

• Drink small sips of water during meals to wash down the flavor of your food.

Early satiety

Early satiety refers to when you feel full sooner than usual when you eat. For example, when you're halfway through a meal, you feel like you can't eat anymore. Early satiety can be caused by stomach surgery, constipation, certain medications, etc.

If you feel full too quickly, try this:

• Eat small, frequent meals.

• Drinking alcohol while eating can help you feel full faster.

• Include high-calorie, high-protein foods in your diet (e.g., low-fat milk powder, wheat germ, nut butters, avocados, oils, butter).

• Do light physical activity (e.g. walking) after eating.

Nausea and vomiting

Nausea means an upset stomach or nausea. Nausea can be caused by radiotherapy, chemotherapy or surgery. Pain, medications, and infections can also cause it.

When you feel nauseous, you may throw up (vomit). If you want to vomit, follow the advice in this section. Stay hydrated with electrolyte-rich drinks. For example, read the Stay Hydrated section of this article.

Below are suggestions for managing nausea through diet. Ask your doctor or nurse if you need antiemetics (medicines to prevent or treat nausea and vomiting).

Fatigue

Fatigue is one of the most common side effects during cancer treatment. This can interfere with normal daily activities. It also affects quality of life and makes treatment harder to tolerate. Fatigue can be caused by a variety of other symptoms, including:

• Loss of appetite

• Depression

• Nausea and vomiting

• Diarrhea or constipation

Managing these symptoms can also help relieve fatigue. Tell your doctor if you have any of the above problems. Another way to control fatigue is to conserve energy, you can:

• On days when you have more energy, make more food. On days when you don't feel like cooking, freeze a portion of food in the freezer for a snack.

• Ways ask family and friends for assistance with shopping and cooking activities.

• Buy ready meals when energy levels are low.

• Keep frequently used ingredients and cooking utensils nearby.

• When cooking, sit instead of standing.

• Eat small, frequent, high-calorie meals or snacks. This way, your body may not need as much energy to digest your food.

Brandon Oliver

CHAPTER 6

THE BEST FOODS TO REDUCE THE RISK OF CANCER

When you think about the dos and don'ts of eating a healthy diet to reduce your cancer risk, it's not a black and white issue. We shouldn't be afraid of food. Instead, take a step back and look at the bigger picture. This allows you to focus on the dietary changes that will have the biggest impact. Some of the best nutrients for cancer prevention and overall healthy living can be found in the Mediterranean diet, which emphasizes whole and plant-based foods. Think more fruits, vegetables, nuts and lean protein and less red meat and prepackaged foods.

Tips to control your weight and reduce the risk of cancer:

Eat more fruits and vegetables

According to the American Cancer Society, eating the rainbow is a good rule of thumb. The pigments that give fruits and vegetables their color contain ingredients that reduce the risk of developing cancer. Try to eat at least three different colored fruits and vegetables every day examples are:

• Red: apples, tomatoes, red cabbage.

• Oranges: melons, carrots, oranges.

• Yellow: banana, lemon, pineapple.

• Vegetables: Broccoli and leafy greens such as spinach, kale and collard greens.

• Blue/grey: beetroot, grapes, blueberries, rhubarb.

These colorful vitamins and minerals all play an important role in cellular health and keeps the body functioning at its best. Try to make potion of your plate fruit and vegetables.

Divide the other half into whole grains, lean meats, fish and plant-based proteins.

Think sugar

When it comes to cancer, some people consider sugar to be public enemy. There is also a saying that sugar feeds cancer. Sugar actually feeds all of our cells, but not all sugar is created equal. The problem is not with foods that contain natural sugars, such as fruit or grains. It is added sugar that causes obesity and heart disease.

When looking at the amount of sugar in your diet, of course there are the usual suspects: sugary drinks, sweets and desserts. But added sugar is also found in many foods that don't scream sugar rush. Hidden sources of sugar include:

• Vessel

• Biscuits

- Muslirepen

- Salad dressing.

- Yogurt, especially fruit-flavored varieties.

To keep your weight in a healthy range and reduce your risk of cancer, keep added sugar low. The American Heart Association recommends no more than 24 grams of added sugar per day for women and those designated as female at birth (AFAB) and no more than 36 grams of added sugar per day for men and those designated as male at birth (AMAB). I recommend doing this.

Consider vitamin D supplements

Low levels of vitamin D have been linked to an increased risk of breast, colon and prostate cancer.

Few foods are naturally rich in vitamin D, but some products, such as soy, almond and oak milk, can be fortified with vitamin D.

Exposure to sunlight (while wearing sunscreen!) can help boost vitamin D, and some people benefit from supplements. Talk to your doctor about whether vitamin D supplements are right for you.

Eat fiber

High-fiber foods keep you full longer, so you don't need to take snack 10 minutes after lunch. Studies have shown that high-fiber foods release acetate, an appetite-suppressing molecule that signals satiety to the brain.

A high-fiber diet is associated with a reduced risk of colon cancer. High-fiber foods are an important addition to a cancer-fighting diet to help control weight because they help you feel full.

Foods high in fiber include:

• Whole grains.

• Beans and lentils.

- Nuts

- Cranberries

Less alcohol

Alcohol consumption has been associated with an increased risk of esophageal, throat, and breast cancer. People who drink a lot of craft beer have a higher risk of developing colorectal cancer. People with alcohol use disorders have a higher risk of liver cancer.

Go easy on the salt

Avoid salty, smoked, and canned foods that contain nitrites, such as sausages, cold cuts, and hot dogs. Studies have shown a high correlation between stomach cancer and high consumption of salty foods.

Cut the fat intake

To control your weight, reduce your daily fat intake, ideally to 25 to 30 grams per day. It's best to be picky with your oil. If you want to continue eating unsaturated fats, look for the words monounsaturated and polyunsaturated fats. Examples of good fats include:

• Almonds (14 g per ounce)

• Findakas (8g per spoon)

• Avocado (10g per half cup)

• Hummus (2g per lingura)

CHAPTER 7

CAN CANCER BE TREATED WITH DIET?

There is no scientific evidence that any diet can cure cancer, but if you are living with cancer, a healthy diet can help:

• The treatment helps the body recover and bounce back.

• Strengthen your immune system.

• Protect healthy cells from environmental damage.

If you have cancer, your doctor can recommend the best diet for you and your condition. We can also discuss your treatment plan and how your diet may affect your cancer. Being flexible about what you eat and how much you eat can help you deal with side effects. While it's important to focus on healthy foods, it's important to avoid unhealthy foods when living with cancer.

Super foods for immune support in cancer patients

Maintaining a strong immune system is important to support the body's ability to fight and heal disease. While no super food guarantees immune support, certain nutrient-dense foods can contribute to overall immune system health. Adding a variety of super foods to your diet can help boost the immune system of cancer patients.

Berries: Berries like blueberries, strawberries, and raspberries are rich in antioxidants, vitamins, and fiber, promote overall immune system health, and help fight oxidative stress.

Citrus fruits: Oranges, grapefruit, lemons and limes are rich in vitamin C, a powerful antioxidant known for its immune-boosting properties.

Ginger: Ginger is known for its anti-inflammatory and antioxidant properties and can help support the immune system. It also helps relieve nausea, a common side effect of cancer treatment.

 Turmeric: Curcumin, the active compound in turmeric, has anti-inflammatory and antioxidant effects and can support the immune system.

Leafy greens: Kale, spinach, Swiss chard, and other dark green leafy vegetables are rich in vitamins, minerals, and antioxidants that benefit your overall health.

Cruciferous vegetables: Broccoli, cauliflower, Brussels sprouts and cabbage contain vitamins, minerals and phytochemicals that support immune function.

Probiotic-Rich Foods: Yogurt, kefir, sauerkraut, and other fermented foods contain probiotics that promote a healthy gut micro biome and immune function.

Nuts and seeds: Almonds, walnuts, chia seeds and flax seeds provide important nutrients like vitamin E and zinc, which are important for immune health.

Fatty fish: Salmon, mackerel and sardines are rich in omega-3 fatty acids, which have anti-inflammatory effects and can support immune function.

Mushrooms: Some mushrooms, such as shiitake and maitake, contain beta-glucans and other compounds that can modulate the immune system.

Green tea: Green tea is rich in antioxidants, including catechins, which may have immune-boosting effects. Sweet potatoes: Sweet potatoes are rich in beta-carotene, which the body converts into vitamin A, which supports immune function.

Protein: Poultry, fish, tofu and legumes provide essential amino acids and nutrients your immune system needs. It is very important for cancer patients to focus on a balanced diet that includes a variety of nutritious foods. However, individual nutritional requirements may vary, so we recommend that you consult a healthcare professional or registered dietitian to tailor nutritional recommendations to each patient's specific situation. In addition, a healthy lifestyle through regular physical activity, adequate sleep and stress management helps with overall immune stability.

Special diet for the special needs of cancer patients

Specialized diets for cancer patients are designed to meet the specific nutritional needs and challenges associated with the disease and treatment. These diets are designed to optimize nutritional intake, support overall health, and manage treatment-related side effects. It is essential to tailor the diet to the individual patient's needs, and health professionals, including registered dietitians, play an important role in developing and monitoring these professional nutritional plans. A common concern is weight loss and malnutrition, which are common in cancer patients. A high-calorie, high-protein diet is often recommended for maintaining or restoring muscle mass and maintaining energy levels. Nutrient-rich foods such as lean protein, whole grains, and healthy fats are important components of this diet.

For people experiencing appetite or taste changes, nutritional strategies may include eating smaller portions more often, emphasizing tasty and appealing foods, and experimenting with different textures and temperatures. You can also add certain foods known for their anti-nausea properties, such as ginger, to ease the nausea associated with the treatment.

People receiving cancer treatment, such as chemotherapy or radiotherapy, may experience changes in their gastrointestinal tract, causing problems such as diarrhea or constipation. In these cases, these symptoms can be controlled by dietary changes, such as increasing fiber to relieve constipation or avoiding certain foods that cause diarrhea.

Additional adjustments may be necessary for patients with special dietary restrictions or pre-existing conditions. For example, people with diabetes must carefully monitor and adjust their carbohydrate intake to control blood sugar levels. People with kidney disease may need to limit certain nutrients, such as potassium and phosphorus. In some cases, certain cancer treatments, surgery, or the location of the tumor can affect your ability to chew or swallow. To address these issues while meeting nutritional requirements, modified textures such as purees or soft foods can be added to the diet. Special diets for cancer patients also take into account the impact of the disease on the immune system. An immune support diet can include foods rich in antioxidants, vitamins and minerals that help strengthen the body's natural defenses. Foods rich in probiotics can be recommended to support gut health, recognizing the important role of the gut micro biome in overall immune function.

Meal plans during a fight against cancer must be flexible and responsive to the individual's changing needs. Regular communication between the patient and the medical staff allows the diet to be adjusted according to the response to treatment, nutritional status and emerging problems.

Practically, special diets for cancer patients are not unique. Rather, it is a customized meal plan designed to meet each person's unique circumstances and needs. These diets are designed to improve overall well-being, manage treatment-related side effects, and promote patient resilience to the complex challenges of cancer.

How to adjust your diet for the different stages of treatment

Dietary modifications for cancer patients at various stages of treatment include adapting nutritional strategies to meet changing needs, managing side effects, and supporting overall well-being. Stages of cancer treatment typically include initial diagnosis, active treatment (e.g. surgery, chemotherapy, or radiation), and post-treatment or survival stages. Below are general guidelines for adjusting the diet at each stage.

Focus on density: Focus on a nutrient-dense diet that includes a variety of fruits, vegetables, whole grains, lean protein, and healthy fats. This helps lay the foundation for optimal health and prepares the body for healing.

Hydration: Encourages adequate hydration. Good hydration is important for your overall health and helps your body tolerate treatment better.

Active treatment (chemotherapy, radiotherapy, surgery)

Calorie and Protein Intake: Address potential weight loss and muscle loss by ensuring adequate calorie and protein intake. Small, frequent meals may be easier for people with loss of appetite or nausea.

Foods that are prone to drying: For patients with digestive problems, include foods that are easily digestible, such as soups, stews and well-cooked vegetables.

Stay hydrated: Some treatments can cause dehydration, so stay hydrated. Encourage drinking water throughout the day and consider hydrating foods such as water-rich fruits.

Control nausea: choose soft, low-fat and easy-to-digest foods. You can add ginger and mint to relieve nausea.

Recovery and Treatment (Survival)

Gradual return to regular diet: Once the patient has completed active treatment, gradually restart another diet.

Manage long-term effects: Manage the long-term side effects of treatment, such as taste changes or persistent digestive problems. A customized meal plan can help solve persistent problems.

Focus on immune support: Focus on immune-supporting foods rich in antioxidants, vitamins and minerals. Include several fruits, grains and vegetables.

Bone health: If necessary, include foods rich in calcium and vitamin D to support bone health, especially if the patient is receiving treatments that affect bone density.

Ongoing Monitoring: Continue to monitor your nutritional status and adjust your diet as needed. Engage in healthy lifestyle, also be part of regular exercise.

Additional considerations

Collaborate with healthcare professionals: Maintain open communication with healthcare professionals every step of the way and involve a registered dietitian to ensure dietary changes are consistent with the patient's overall treatment plan.

Personalized Planning: We recognize each patient's unique needs and preferences. Adjust your diet based on your individual response to treatment, side effects, and existing medical conditions. Adapting diet to the different stages of cancer treatment is a dynamic process that requires flexibility and continuous evaluation. By tailoring nutrition to the specific needs of the patient at each stage, healthcare providers can improve overall outcomes and improve the quality of life of people receiving cancer treatment.

CHAPTER 8

COOKING METHOD THAT HELPS CANCER PATIENTS DIGEST FOOD EASILY

Cooking for cancer patients often involves applying methods to improve the digestibility of food, especially for patients with digestive problems or treatment-related side effects. The cooking methods that help the digestion of cancer patients are as follows:

Steaming: Steaming is a gentle cooking method that preserves the natural moisture in food. Suitable for vegetables, fish and poultry. steamed food is very easy to digest.

Poaching: Poaching involves cooking food in boiling liquid. This method is often used for delicate proteins such as fish or eggs. The low temperature and humidity help to maintain the softness.

Slow cooking: Slow cooking, whether using a pot or a slow cooker, means cooking food at a low temperature for a long time. This method can be helpful in breaking down tough meat fibers and making them easier to chew and digest.

Blending and pureeing: Blending and pureeing food can help people who have difficulty chewing or swallowing. Soups, smoothies and vegetable purees have a smooth texture that makes them easier on the digestive system.

Mashing: Pureeing is a simple method for vegetables, fruits and cooked beans. It creates a soft texture, making food tastier and easier to digest.

Grilling and barbecuing: During grilling and grilling, the fat drips from the meat, making it thinner. However, overcooking or burning the pieces should be avoided as this can damage the digestive system.

Cooking: Cooking is a versatile method that can be used in a variety of dishes. Useful in low protein dishes, vegetables and fruits. Choose tender cuts of meat and add liquid if necessary.

Sautéing with healthy fats: Sauteing vegetables and lean proteins with a small amount of healthy fats, such as olive oil or canola oil, improves flavor and digestibility. Use as little oil as possible to avoid excessive oil consumption.

Marinating: Marinating meat before cooking tenderizes it and adds flavor. Using a slightly acidic marinade that contains herbs and spices can enhance flavor without causing digestive discomfort.

 Use strong flavors and spices: People with sensitive palates or stomachs may find it helpful to limit their use of strong flavors and spices. Choose mild spices and herbs.

Texture Adjustment: Adjust the texture of food based on personal tastes and tolerances. For example, some people prefer their vegetables finely chopped, while others prefer a pureed texture. Moisture during cooking: Adding moisture to dishes, such as by using stock or adding sauces, prevents dehydration and enhances the flavor of the dish.

Small, frequent meals: Eating small, frequent meals instead of large meals can ease the digestive system, especially in people with loss of appetite or nausea.

 Individual approach: consider personal preferences and food tolerance. Talk to the person receiving the treatment to understand their specific needs and adjust your cooking methods accordingly. It is important to consult with a health care professional, including a registered dietitian, to develop a personalized nutrition plan that meets the unique needs of each cancer patient. Adapting cooking methods to personal preferences and digestive comfort can contribute to an enjoyable and nutritious cooking experience during cancer treatment.

Tips for preparing soft, easy-to-swallow foods for cancer patients

Preparing foods that are soft and easy to swallow is especially important for cancer patients who may have trouble chewing, swallowing, or other digestive problems related to their disease or treatment. Below is more information on preparing these dishes:

1. **Choose soft textures:** Choose soft textures that are easy to chew and swallow, such as cooked vegetables, tender meats and soft grains.

2. **Cooking techniques**

Steaming: Steaming vegetables and proteins retains moisture and makes them tender.

Cooking: Cook the vegetables, pasta or rice until soft. Cooking: Cook or grill the meat using broiled until it is tender and pulls apart easily.

Slow Cooker: Whether you're making stews, soups, casseroles, and more, a slow cooker can help you create tender, well-cooked meals.

 3. Puree and Gluttony: Puree or blend food to create a smooth texture suitable for people who have difficulty chewing or swallowing. Soups, smoothies and vegetable purees are good choices.

4. Soft proteins: choose lean meat and poultry. Ground meat, buns, and shredded chicken or turkey are easier to manage. Eat protein sources such as tofu, eggs and fish that can be cooked to a soft texture.

5. Making and breaking: Vegetables such as potatoes, sweet potatoes, carrots and beans are mashed to create a smooth, easily digestible consistency. You can make many dishes creamier by adding mashed avocado or banana.

6. Dairy Substitutes: Use dairy alternatives such as yogurt, milk or non-dairy milk in smoothies, soups or as a sauce base to add a nutritious and smooth texture.

7. Casseroles and One-Pot Dishes: Make casseroles or one-pot dishes that combine multiple ingredients into one smooth, cohesive dish.

8. Applesauce and fruit purees: As a natural sweetener, add applesauce or other fruit purees to baked goods or sauces for an extra source of moisture.

9. Avoid hard or fiber-rich foods: Avoid hard, crunchy or fibrous foods that can be difficult to chew or swallow. These include raw vegetables, nuts and hard meats.

10. Soups and broths: Make nutritious soups and broths with well-cooked vegetables, lean proteins, and bland grains. It's easy to drink and keeps you hydrated.

11. Egg-based dishes: Eggs are a versatile and mild source of protein. Try making scrambled eggs, scrambled eggs or casseroles.

12. Herbs and herbal adjustments: Consider your personal tastes and sensitivities. Adjust spices and seasonings to account for changes in taste or sensitivity to certain flavors.

13. Moisturizing foods: Add moisture to foods by adding sauces, gravies, or soups. This can improve both taste and ease of swallowing.

14. Personal preferences: Consider your personal preferences and get feedback from the person receiving the treatment. Encourage children to talk about the textures, tastes and temperatures of their favorite foods.

15. Nutrient Density: Prioritize nutrient-dense foods to ensure all foods contain essential vitamins, minerals and calories.

16. Small Meals: Instead of large meals, eat smaller, more frequent meals throughout the day to prevent fatigue and ensure you're getting enough nutrients.

17. Collaborate with a dietitian: Work closely with a registered dietitian to develop a customized meal plan based on your specific needs and preferences. Adapting cooking methods and preparing delicate, easy-to-swallow foods requires creativity and flexibility. The goal is to support the nutritional needs of cancer patients while providing nutritious and attractive options for those who have difficulty chewing or swallowing. Regular communication with health professionals and the person receiving treatment allows the diet to be adapted to the patient's changing needs and preferences.

Obstacles to diet change and how to overcome them

Changing eating habits is difficult. Even with good intentions, it can be difficult to replace unhealthy foods with healthy eating habits.

If you're having trouble eating well, you may be facing one of these common obstacles:

Lack of time

Like anything you want to achieve, you need to have a healthy eating plan. Set aside time in your calendar for meal planning, shopping, and prep so you can find healthy foods on hand.

You can also use time-saving tricks like buying pre-cut produce, using a slow cooker, or doubling recipes to ensure you have leftovers that can be frozen. Keep a list of quick and healthy meals and snacks to avoid confusion when shopping and cooking. You can also buy groceries online to save time.

Feeling of connection

Don't try to make too many changes at once. Over time, small changes can have a big impact, and it's much cheaper. Difficult change can be both overwhelming and difficult to manage, leading to feelings of self-doubt.

Mastering small changes will build your confidence and small improvements will become part of your lifestyle. Once you've established a new habit, start another. Change is a process, not an event.

An all or nothing attitude

If you decide to change your eating habits, you may feel like you have no room for error. At some point you will experience repetitions and frustrations. If you have an all-or-nothing mentality, failure can feel like failure and cause you to give up.

Remember, you're aiming for progress, not perfection. Treat failure as an obstacle and keep moving forward. Change takes time, but if you keep at it, you will achieve your goals.

Diet confusion

With the abundance of fad diets and all the sources of nutritional information, making healthy eating decisions can be difficult and confusing. This can lead to trying different diets and following nutritional advice that is not based on facts. A registered dietitian can help dispel misinformation and provide healthy eating recommendations that work for you and your lifestyle. A nutritionist can also provide ongoing support, accountability and encouragement.

Feeling deprived

Starting a healthier lifestyle may mean giving up some of your favorite foods. But eating healthy doesn't mean you have to say goodbye to all your favorite foods. All foods can be accommodated. Eating well means learning how to eat a variety of foods in moderation. A nutritionist can help you learn how to balance the foods you like with other foods so you can maintain a healthy weight and reduce your risk of chronic disease.

CHAPTER 9

LOW SUGAR AND LOW-FAT VARIATIONS FOR CANCER PATIENTS

Creating low-sugar and low-fat options for cancer patients requires a careful approach to meet nutritional needs, manage potential side effects, and support overall wellness. These changes are designed to provide a delicious and satisfying option when addressing the nutritional challenges associated with cancer and its treatment.

Instructions for sugar

Choose fruit: Choose fresh or frozen fruit that is low in natural sugars. Berries, cantaloupes and citrus can add sweetness without adding too much sugar. Experiment with common parts of fruit like apples, pears and peaches and consider baking or grilling them for better flavor.

Natural sweeteners: Choose low-glycemic natural sweeteners in moderation, such as honey, maple syrup, or agave juice. For added sugar-free sweetness, look for sugar substitutes like stevia or monk fruit.

Whole grains: Choosing whole grains like quinoa, barley, and oats over refined grains can give you long-lasting energy without a spike in blood sugar.

Balanced snacking: The combination of protein and fiber helps stabilize blood sugar levels in the snack. For example, nut butter with apple slices or yogurt with a few nuts.

Portion Control: Emphasizes portion control to manage total carbohydrate intake. Eating smaller, more frequent meals can help you maintain your energy levels without putting too much strain on your body.

Limit processed foods: Minimize your consumption of processed foods that contain hidden sugars. To better control added sugars, choose whole, unprocessed foods.

Drink Monitor: Watch out for sugary drinks. Choose water, herbal teas and infused waters rather than sugary soft drinks or fruit juices.

Low fat nutrition

Lean protein: Choose lean protein sources such as skinless poultry, fish, beans and tofu. Provides essential nutrients without excess fat.

Healthy fats: Eat healthy fats in moderation, such as avocados, nuts, seeds and olive oil. Promotes satiety and provides essential nutrients.

Grilling and baking: Choose cooking methods that use less oil, such as grilling, grilling or frying. These methods enhance flavor without relying heavily on oil or fat.

Low-fat or reduced-fat dairy products: Choose low-fat or reduced-fat dairy products such as milk, yogurt and cheese to reduce your overall fat intake while getting calcium and other important nutrients.

Limit saturated and trans fats: Reduce your intake of saturated and trans fats found in fried foods, processed foods, and some baked goods. These fats can cause inflammation and other health problems.

Light salad dressing: Choose a light salad dressing with an olive oil and vinegar vinaigrette or a homemade salad dressing. It reduces the amount of saturated fat and improves the taste.

Steam and bake: Reduce added fat and preserve nutritional value by steaming or baking vegetables instead of roasting or grilling them.

Read the labels: Read food labels to discover hidden fats and make informed choices. Look for products that are low in saturated and trans fats.

Use low-sugar and low-fat strategies

Delicious herbs and spices: Use herbs, spices and citrus fruits to enhance the flavor of low-sugar, low-fat foods. These additives add flavor without relying on excess sugar or fat.

Balanced Meals: Create balanced meals with a mix of lean proteins, whole grains and colorful vegetables to ensure balanced nutrition.

Personalized Plan: Work with a healthcare professional or registered dietitian to create a personalized meal plan that meets each patient's unique needs, taking into account specific treatment response and dietary preferences.

Creating low-sugar and low-fat variations for cancer patients requires creativity, nutritional knowledge, and attention to personal preferences. These changes are designed to provide nutritious and delicious options that promote overall wellness during the challenging journey of cancer treatment.

Strengthening cancer patients through nutrition

Living with cancer is often a difficult experience. You may face various obstacles of a physical, psychological and emotional nature. One of the keys to navigating this is having an effective toolkit. Not only is it a practical way to solve a problem, but it can also help you take more control of your own well-being. These tools can take many forms. Of course, the medications and treatments you take can affect your health. You can also see a therapist or counselor who can show you strategies for managing the psychological symptoms you're experiencing. However, one of the most important factors affecting your daily well-being is your food choices.

CHAPTER 10

IMPROVES OVERALL HEALTH

The experiences of cancer patients can vary. However, it's important to pay attention to your overall health and well-being to be in the best position to deal with the challenges that come with a diagnosis. Nourishing the body and mind plays an important role here.

Of course, this also includes maintaining a balanced diet. Fruits, vegetables, poultry, fish and nuts can be important in promoting your health if you have cancer. Protein sources such as eggs, seeds and lentils contribute to a strong immune system. You should also focus on staying hydrated by drinking water regularly.

In addition to balancing the healthy foods you consume in your body, you should also avoid foods and drinks that can have negative consequences. Alcohol, in particular, can have short-term and long-term negative health effects. Effects on the central nervous system can contribute to or worsen mood swings, and chronic alcohol consumption can cause immune deficiencies. Therefore, if you are undergoing cancer treatment, it may be more beneficial to reduce or significantly reduce your alcohol consumption.

Use of substitutes and supplements

It is not always practical for cancer patients to obtain nutrients directly from food. This is especially important if your treatment affects your appetite. It is worth noting that some drugs, such as chemotherapy, can deplete certain proteins and vitamins stored in the body. It's important to consider how specific supplements and dietary changes can fill any gaps in your nutritional needs.

If you are undergoing cancer treatment, it is important to be careful when adding supplements to your diet. Choose a goal-oriented approach. Discuss with your oncology team which vitamins you are deficient in and which may have a strengthening or protective effect. You should also be aware that some supplements can harm the effectiveness of your treatment. For example, plant compounds such as garlic, ginseng, and echinacea can interfere with the body's metabolism of chemotherapy drugs. Therefore, do not make any changes without the advice of a specialist.

A good approach to your diet is to find substitutes for foods that are hard to digest or generally unhealthy. For example, even if you crave sweet treats, processed sugar can harm your cognition, mood, and overall well-being. It's usually best to find alternatives in the form of healthy, naturally sweet foods like fruit, nuts and homemade snacks. This can be a useful strategy when dealing with treatment issues. Not to mention, natural foods taste better when you're nauseous.

Mitigating treatment side-effects

Navigating the truth about cancer can be difficult. While therapy is a powerful tool for healing and recovery, it can also impact the challenges you face. The side effects of radiotherapy, chemotherapy and many other factors can affect your quality of life. It's worth exploring how your food choices can help with this problem. Changes in appetite and nausea are among the most common side effects of cancer treatment. A healthy approach to this is to consume smoothies instead of solid foods. It eases digestion and helps you get the fruits and vegetables you need.

In addition, some cancer patients wake up with diarrhea and other bowel or bladder problems as a result of their treatment. It is best to avoid fried, spicy or fatty foods, especially in the first few days after treatment. You can follow a pure liquid diet that includes broth, gelatin and some fruit juices. Bananas and potatoes can also be a positive replacement for some of the potassium you may lose through diarrhea.

Brandon Oliver

CONCLUSION

It's not just about closing the book. The most important thing is to enjoy the journey shared through these pages. Think of it as the lingering taste of satisfying, warming, satisfying comfort food.

Our culinary adventures have us stirring pots, testing flavors, and creating dishes that are more than just recipes. This is a story of care and resilience. From silky textures to low-sugar and low-fat options, we've created each dish with the unique challenge of fighting cancer in mind.

But this is not just a cookbook. Your friend and companion encourage you as you embrace the healing power of food. Cooking here is not a chore. This is an act of healing that reminds us that the kitchen can be a place of joy and strength, even in difficult times.

As we close this page, don't forget the essence of what we do. It is more than materials and technology. It's about the conversations shared the laughter in the kitchen and the warmth that a well-prepared meal brings to the table.

For every reader, caregiver, or warrior fighting cancer, consider this cookbook a gift that will give you a warm hug in the kitchen. I hope this recipe will continue to be a source of comfort, nourishment and joy for you and your loved ones. The kitchen is a space and sanctuary for creation, healing and celebration. Use these recipes in your own culinary adventures, allowing each dish to reflect your inner strength and resilience. Introducing the good food, health and warm moments that come from sharing food. Cheers to you!

Brandon Oliver